CBD

Heal Naturally Without Drugs

The Advanced Guide
For Medicinal Cannabis
To Improve Health &
Reduce Pain

© **Copyright 2018 by Dr. J Arthur - All rights reserved.**

This document is geared towards providing exact and reliable information in regards to the topic and issue covered. The publication is sold with the idea that the publisher is not required to render accounting, officially permitted, or otherwise, qualified services. If advice is necessary, legal or professional, a practiced individual in the profession should be ordered.

- From a Declaration of Principles which was accepted and approved equally by a Committee of the American Bar Association and a Committee of Publishers and Associations.

In no way is it legal to reproduce, duplicate, or transmit any part of this document by either electronic means or in printed format. Recording of this publication is strictly prohibited and any storage of this document is not allowed unless with written permission from the publisher. All rights reserved.

The information provided herein is stated to be truthful and consistent, in that any liability, in terms of inattention or otherwise, by any usage or abuse of any policies, processes, or directions contained within is the solitary and utter responsibility of the recipient reader. Under no circumstances will any legal responsibility or blame be held against the publisher for any reparation, damages, or monetary loss due to the information herein, either directly or indirectly.

Respective authors own all copyrights not held by the publisher.

The information herein is offered for informational purposes solely and is universal as so. The presentation of the information is without a contract or any type of guarantee assurance.

The trademarks that are used are without any consent, and the publication of the trademark is without permission or backing by the trademark owner. All trademarks and brands within this book are for clarifying purposes only and are the owned by the owners themselves, not affiliated with this document.

Table of Contents

Introduction

Chapter One: Cannabidiol (CBD)

    What is Cannabinoid?

    What is Cannabidiol?

    Where can you find Cannabidiol?

Chapter Two: History of Cannabis

    History of the pot

        Medical Cannabis

        Weed for recreational purpose

    CBD – Hemp or Marijuana!

    Cannabis legalization and the Marijuana Tax Act

Chapter Three: How Does the Medical Cannabis Work?

    How does this magic weed work?

        Endogenous cannabinoids

        Cannabinoid Receptors

- When plant cannabinoids meet endocannabinoid
- Restoring the balance
- Does CBD work for recreational purposes similar to THC?
- Is Cannabidiol the future of healing?
  - Medical Cannabis and the diseases it can help treat

Chapter Four: How to Use?

- THC and CBD – the better element
- Best ways to consume CBD
  - Different ways to consume CBD
  - Ingest CBD
  - Hold under the tongue
  - Vaping
  - Chew as a gum
  - Mix with your food or drink
  - Apply Topically
  - Wash or condition hair using CBD

Chapter Five: CBD for Chronic Pain

- Chronic pain relief
  - Multiple sclerosis
  - Generic acute pain
- Dosage, Side effects, and Benefits
- Studies and Researches

Chapter Six: Anxiety and Seizures

- Anxiety
- How CBD reduces anxiety?
- Seizures
- More Studies and Researches

Chapter Seven: Fibromyalgia

- Effect of CBD on Fibromyalgia pain
- Studies and Researches

Chapter Eight: CBD to Reduce Opioids

- Role of cannabis in Opioids and Chronic Pain
  - Block the addiction
- Case Study

- Inference

Chapter Nine: CBD for Cancer

- Does CBD fight the cancer cells?
  - Things to remember
- Clinical trials
  - Cancer
  - Chemotherapy

Chapter Ten: CBD for Health

- How does CBD promote to improve health?
- Dietary necessities provided by CBD

Chapter Eleven: Safety and Legal Issues

- Difference between Legal and Illegal CBD oil

Conclusion

Sources

Introduction

I want to thank you for purchasing this book: *"CBD Heal Naturally Without Drugs"*

Popping pills has become extremely common; it is alarming how many people depend on pills. People take medicines (mostly self-medication) for everything from a simple headache to the deadliest disease. Curing the ailment is one thing, but the side effects caused by the treatment are sometimes disturbing. Almost all the medicines we use have positives and negatives to them – but, of late, the negatives seem to be on the higher end. Antibiotics, painkillers, sleeping pills, etc. – are said to have serious or not-so-serious side effects.

Wouldn't it be good if we could heal our minds and bodies the natural way? Nature has already given us whatever is needed to survive and live on this planet in harmony. Unfortunately, we humans are so busy running the race of life that we don't stop for a moment to look around us. If we look around, the answer is always found in nature.

The magic herb, Cannabis, is one such element found in nature that works in a wonderful manner. It can help heal illness and improve wellness without depending on chemicals and pills. Medical marijuana, also known as medical cannabis, is said to provide a lot of solutions. Cannabidiol (CBD), one of the main molecules, present in this magic herb (marijuana) can heal the human body from a lot of chronic and deadly diseases. Apart from marijuana, CBD can also be derived from the industrial hemp plant.

Is there a difference between marijuana and industrial hemp? Not really!

Scientifically speaking, Marijuana and industrial hemp are the same plants of the genus *Cannabis Sativa*. They have a different genetic profile. It is more about how these plants are bred that differentiates them. Marijuana will be smaller and bushier while industrial hemp will be fibrous with longer stalks. The composition of the CBD component in these plants also makes a difference. Marijuana has less CBD and more THC (another cannabinoid molecule) while industrial hemp has more CBD and less THC. If the THC component is more in the herb, consuming the product can make you feel high. This is why you get high when you consume marijuana, but not with hemp.

This book will act as a beginner's guide to anyone who would like to use medicinal cannabis for pain management. The chapters will concentrate on what CBD is, the history of cannabis, the effect it can have on the human body and the benefits it holds.

By the time you finish with this book, you will be more confident and ready to give this magic herb a serious try!

I hope this book serves as an interesting and informative read. Happy reading!

Chapter One: Cannabidiol (CBD)

Cannabidiol (CBD) is one of the many molecular components found naturally in cannabis and the industrial hemp plant. This particular component is a non-psychoactive cannabinoid that is found in cannabis (popularly known as marijuana). Since this component is the key to healing many medical conditions, more research and studies are conducted on the effective usage of cannabis. The CBD component in cannabis can cure a variety of medical conditions without getting you high.

What is Cannabinoid?

This is a class of chemical compound that acts on the cannabinoid receptors in the body cells. This is responsible for altering the release of neurotransmitters in the human brain. Our human body has cannabinoid receptors that get disturbed when an external cannabinoid (in marijuana or hemp) reacts with it. There are close to 100 plus cannabinoids identified in cannabis.

Tetrahydrocannabinol or THC is another cannabinoid, which is found in cannabis along with other cannabinoids. This is similar to CBD, but the only difference between the two is CBD in non-psychoactive while THC is psychoactive. This principal psychoactive constituent of cannabis is the reason why you get high when you consume marijuana.

The cannabis plants are chemical powerhouses that can produce 400 plus different compounds. Out of these 400 compounds, almost 60 are specific only to Cannabis (plant genus) and will not be found in any other plant species. These special compounds were named cannabinoids by scientists. It is essential to understand that not all cannabinoids are created equal – each of them has their own properties. CBD is one cannabinoid, which has numerous medicinal properties.

Marijuana usually has a low amount of CBD and a high amount of THC (99 percent of the time). But when you look at the industrial hemp plant, it is vice-versa. The plant naturally has a high amount of CBD and only traces of THC in most instances. People who want to enjoy the benefits of cannabis without getting high can choose the cannabinoid profile of industrial hemp. Hemp is used to make fiber, paper, bricks, oil, herbal supplements, rope, natural plastic, food and many more products. But marijuana is specifically used for recreational, medicinal and spiritual purpose.

Cannabis oil can be made either from industrial hemp or marijuana, as both are two different cannabis forms. Irrespective of the plant (marijuana or hemp) it is made from, CBD is the same (there is no major difference apart for the composition of the component). Apart from CBD, there are many other non-psychoactive cannabinoid components, such as, CBG (Cannabigerol), CBC (Cannabichromene), etc. found in cannabis plants. Marijuana (cannabis) has the lowest non-psychoactive cannabinoids.

What is Cannabidiol?

Cannabidiol (CBD) is the non-psychoactive cannabinoid found in cannabis (marijuana) and industrial hemp. This natural chemical component has considerable medical benefits that can counteract with the psychoactive component in THC. While the THC component can make you feel stoned, CBD works otherwise. CBD-rich cannabis is an alluring option for patients who want to ease their pain or for relief from anxiety, inflammation, seizures, psychosis, spasms and many other severe medical conditions. The non-psychoactive component or the less psychoactive composition, when compared to the strains rich in THC doesn't give the unsettled feeling of uneasiness or lethargy.

CBD is one of the cannabinoid components in Cannabis, which is found in abundance after THC. This plant-derived cannabinoid, also known as phytocannabinoid, can act with the cannabinoid receptors that are part of our endocannabinoid system. Though THC also has certain medicinal uses, it is CBD that tops the chart with its broad range of potential medical benefits. And the best part is it heals the body and mind without getting you into an intoxicated state. This makes CBD a therapeutic agent.

Cannabinoids are growing popular on a global scale as a breakthrough wellness supplement and nutritional component. After enough media coverage on CBD's miraculous benefits, it has become a household name enabling more and more people to try it for health and wellness.

More clinical and scientific research has proved that CBD is a potential natural medicine to treat a variety of medical conditions such as:

- Depression
- Epilepsy
- Neurological disorders
- PTSD
- Chronic pain

- Arthritis
- Alcoholic-addiction
- Diabetes
- Schizophrenia
- Antibiotic-resistant infections

It is said that CBD has potential neurogenic and Neuroprotective effects. Many research centers in the United States are trying to find more about its anti-cancer properties. CBD can be found in the flowers, stalks, and seeds of the cannabis plants. Most of the time, this non-psychoactive cannabinoid is extracted from the plants in the form of cannabis oil.

Where can you find Cannabidiol?

As mentioned earlier, Cannabidiol (CBD) is most commonly found in cannabis (marijuana) plant. However, that is not the only source of CBD. CBD can be produced in different ways:

- The natural source of CBD is obviously the cannabis plant. The plant will first create the cannabigerolic acid (CBGa). This compound will then be used by the plant to create the cannabidiolic acid (CBDa). CBDa then gets decarboxylated (loses the carboxyl group) to CBD due to various factors such as time, light or heat. When the acid form (CBDa) loses carbon dioxide (CO_2), it becomes CBD.

- Similarly, CBGa can be maneuvered by the cannabis plant to create THCa (tetrahydrocannabinolic acid). On losing the carbon dioxide (CO_2), it becomes THC.
- CBD can also be produced in a laboratory synthetically. Even if the cannabinoid is produced synthetically, possessing it (except under specific circumstances) is still considered illegal, as it is a regulated substance.

CBD is found in both varieties of cannabis – hemp and marijuana. The level of THC is the only difference that is to be noted in both these plants. Marijuana grown for recreational purpose specifically contains a high level of THC whereas hemp will only have traces of THC.

Our human body also creates a Cannabidiol-like molecule (2-Arachidonyglycerol or 2-AG) naturally. This endocannabinoid has similar neuromodulatory effects as CBD and therefore, acts as an agonist to the CB1 receptor (cannabinoid type-1 receptor found in the central nervous system). The 2-AG has been detected in the human breast milk.

The more you learn about CBD and its therapeutic benefits, the more surprised you will be!

Chapter Two: History of Cannabis

Humans have used cannabis, popularly known as pot or marijuana, for quite a long time (since ancient days!). Primitive people cultivated the plant around 500 BC to use it as herbal medicine. It started with Asian cultures initially. The early colonists in America were involved in cannabis cultivation for the production of rope and textiles. They grew hemp for various other needs during the early days. But with racial and political factors building up, the United States officially termed the use of cannabis (marijuana) as a criminal offense in the 20th century. It is only recently that the status is changing in places across the country.

The origin of hemp or cannabis plant is said to be from Central Asia before it was introduced to Europe, Africa and finally the United States. The fiber from the hemp plant was mostly used for the production of paper, rope, clothes, sails, etc. They used the hemp seeds as food. The history of cannabis is said to have started from the time primeval hunters and gatherers. These people mostly used the plant for spiritual and medicinal purposes. For instance, the medieval Germans and the Vikings used cannabis to relieve pain during childbirth. They had also used it for toothaches.

Since this plant grows fast, it was cultivated all through colonial America and in the Southwest Spanish region. It was in the early 1600s when few colonies in Massachusetts, Connecticut, and Virginia were looking for farmers to grow the hemp plant. The hemp plants grown in those days had very low traces of THC. Few evidences pointed out that many ancient cultures had in fact known about the psychoactive properties of the cannabis plant. It is believed that they might have grown few varieties of cannabis plants that produce high THC levels and used them for spiritual practices. Burned cannabis seeds (which dates back to 500 BC) were found in the shaman graves in Siberia and China.

An old written record confirms the usage of Cannabis by the Chinese Emperor Shen Nung in 2727 BC. Romans and Greeks also used Cannabis in the ancient days after which it slowly spread to the Middle East and North Africa. The Spaniards imported Cannabis to Chile in 1545 for fiber usage. Later it was grown in North America in the form of hemp for production of paper, rope, and clothing.

Currently, the plant *Cannabis Sativa* is found in many humid and tropical parts of the world. The seeds are used for feeding animals, the fiber for hemp rope and the oil for paint. This plant is dioeciously, which produces male and female plant. The tall, thin plants with flower-like pods are male. Their pods contain the anthers that generate pollens for fertilization. The female plants are shorter and darker with tiny hairs protruding at the end of the bracteole pods.

History of the pot

Before studying the history, it is crucial to understand the difference between the subspecies of the cannabis plants. The *Cannabis Sativa,* also known as marijuana or cannabis, has psychoactive properties while the other subspecies *Cannabis Sativa L,* also known as hemp, has non-psychoactive properties. The L in *Cannabis Sativa L* was referred to honor Carl Linnaeus, the botanist who introduced the binomial nomenclature in plant organisms. The hemp plant is mostly used for manufacturing fuel, cloth, and oil.

Apart from these two cannabis plants, two other plants were identified for their psychoactive properties. Jean Baptiste Lamarck, a French Naturalist, introduced another subspecies of cannabis plant known as *Cannabis Indica*. D.E. Janischevisky, a Russian botanist, had introduced the third but uncommon psychoactive species of cannabis plant known as *Cannabis Ruderalis*. Most of the cannabis plants are believed to have evolved wildly on a large area of flat non-forested grasslands in Central Asia. These regions are now Southern Siberia and Mongolia.

The cannabis plant has a 12000-year-old history, which makes it the oldest cultivated crops of humankind. Dr. Barney Warf, an expert in Cannabis, says - "*It likely flourished in the nutrient-rich dump sites of prehistoric hunters and gatherers,*"

They found charred cannabis seeds in the burial mounds of Kurgan in Siberia, dated back to 3000 BC. Graves of noble families in Xinjiang, China had large amounts of marijuana in a mummified state, which dates back to 2500 BC. This marijuana was psychoactive. Ancient China used both psychoactive marijuana as well as hemp. The plant is used as a medicinal drug in 4000 BC. It was used for anesthesia in surgeries.

Medical Cannabis

An Irish doctor by the name Sir William Brooke O'Shaughnessy, who was studying in India in the 1830s, found medicinal properties in Cannabis. He was able to prove that extract of the cannabis plant can help reduce vomiting and stomachache in people who suffered from Cholera. After this, pharmacies and clinics started selling cannabis extracts throughout the US and Europe for stomach-related treatments. This happened around the late 1800s.

It was later found that the medicinal properties in cannabis (marijuana) were due to the THC component. This psychoactive compound was responsible for the mind-altering effects caused by Marijuana. THC is said to interact with the areas of the brain to increase appetite and reduce nausea.

The US Food and Drug Administration has approved THC in two drugs – Syndros and Marinol in pill format. They are used to treat loss of appetite in AIDS patients and nausea caused by chemotherapy in cancer patients.

Weed for recreational purpose

A Greek historian, Herodotus, mentioned that Scythians used the Cannabis flowers and seeds to get high. These Iranian nomads in Central Asia (Scythians) consumed Cannabis in the form of smoke. Around 800 AD, Hashish was used in parts of Asia and throughout the Middle East for recreational purpose. Hashish is a purified cannabis form, smoked with a pipe. This became popular across regions where the spread of Islam religion was prevalent. The Quran does not specifically prohibit the use of cannabis like it does for alcohol and other intoxicating stuff.

Till early 1900, marijuana was strictly used for medicinal purpose in the United States. It was only after the Mexicans migrated to the United States during the tumultuous years of Mexican Revolution, things changed. The practice of smoking marijuana for recreational purpose was introduced to the American culture. Social unrest and massive unemployment had forced people to show bitterness towards the Mexican immigrants (as they were the ones who introduced marijuana as an intoxicating substance). It was during the Great Depression in the United States that marijuana was termed as the *evil weed*. This resulted in its Prohibition in the United States, which led to a nationwide ban on all alcoholic products. By the end of 1931, around 29 states had banned the use of cannabis completely.

CBD – Hemp or Marijuana!

Marijuana and hemp plants are two major sources of Cannabidiol (CBD). The legal status of CBD made from cannabis depends on the legal status of marijuana in that particular state in the US. The THC levels in the CBD product determines if the said product is legal or not (especially if medical marijuana is illegal in the particular state). CBD products made from hemp plants are completely legal. But if CBD is derived from marijuana, then the composition of THC should be less than one percent or as low as 0.3 percent for that product to be considered legal.

The fact is, CBD derived from marijuana is said to be more effective and potent when compared to the ones made from the hemp plant. This is because of the entourage effect (when a cannabinoid works together with its companion cannabinoids, it can do its job better). When Cannabidiol (CBD) is extracted from cannabis (marijuana) flowers, it helps to keep the other cannabinoids together. The cannabis plant buds have a richer complement of cannabinoids compared to the leaves of the hemp plant. This is the main reason for people to prefer cannabis-derived CBD to hemp-derived CBD.

After the extraction of cannabis oil, the cannabis industry uses the CBD to process various commercial products in the form of capsules, liquids, etc. They also further isolate CBD from the oil by purifying it to its crystalline form. The CBD products that are made from cannabis oil can be found in wellness stores, medical marijuana dispensaries and online retailers.

CBD products derived from hemp plants are legal in the United States while CBD products made from cannabis (marijuana) are federally illegal. Most of the states in the country are gradually legalizing the usage of marijuana for medicinal purpose. As per Section 7606 of the Agricultural Appropriations Act of 2014, industrial hemp is defined as,

"The term "industrial hemp" means the plant Cannabis sativa L. and any part of such plant, whether growing or not, with a delta-9 Tetrahydrocannabinol concentration of not more than 0.3 percent on a dry weight basis."

Cannabis strain or products, which have more CBD than THC or equal amount of CBD and THC, are referred as CBD-rich products. If the cannabis strains have more CBD and less THC, it is referred as CBD dominant products.

Cannabis legalization and the Marijuana Tax Act

The first federate US law to criminalize marijuana nationwide happened in 1937. The Marijuana Tax Act levied an excise tax on all the hemp products (possession, sales, and cultivation). The law allowed only industrial uses of the hemp plant. Samuel Caldwell became the first individual to get arrested under this act for the sale of marijuana. The 58-year-old farmer was convicted the next day after the act was passed.

Industrial hemp was cultivated across the United States all through the World War II. When the Philippines fell into the hands of the Japanese army, domestic cultivation of the hemp plant was encouraged all over the country. The Philippines was the major source of imported hemp fiber. Wisconsin had its last US hemp fields planted in 1957.

President Richard Nixon signed the law, which listed Marijuana as a Schedule I drug with no medicinal use, under the Controlled Substance Act of 1970. Marijuana was considered to have the same harmful effects as ecstasy, heroin, and LSD. Later, a report titled *Marijuana: A Signal of Misunderstanding* was released by the Shafer Commission (National Commission on Marijuana and Drug Abuse) in 1972. The report recommended lower penalties for possessing small amounts of cannabis and its partial prohibition. But the report's findings were completely ignored by President Nixon and the government authorities.

The first state to legalize cannabis for medicinal use was California. The Compassionate Use Act of 1996 allowed people with chronic illnesses to use medicinal marijuana. Today, Washington DC and nine other states have legalized the use of marijuana for recreational purpose. The US territories of Puerto Rico and Guam, Washington DC and twenty-nine states have legalized the use of cannabis for medicinal purposes. You can use cannabis without a medical prescription in Oregon, Nevada, Maine, Alaska, California, Massachusetts, and Vermont.

Though Cannabis is still illegal under the United States Federal law, the growing popularity of the legality of marijuana is still a subject of controversy around the globe.

Chapter Three: How Does the Medical Cannabis Work?

The network of neurons that runs throughout the body is the major reason for all the cannabinoids unique to the plant genus *Cannabis,* to interact with the human body. This super cool network of neurons is called the endocannabinoid system. This system has numerous receptors that bind to the plant cannabinoids that are introduced into your bloodstream when you consume cannabis (marijuana). The chemical interactions that happen when the cannabinoids bind with the receptors create a series of responses in the human body.

The endocannabinoid system is responsible for the major functionalities of the human body, making cannabis beneficial to us in many ways. Humans are hard-wired for weed! Consuming weed in the right quantity can alter and regulate moods, reduce chronic pain, stimulate appetite, etc. The Cannabidiol (CBD) in the weed is highly reactive with the endocannabinoid system of the body. CBD can stimulate all kinds of changes in the body when it binds to the receptors of the endocannabinoid system. In short, CBD can make things work better! Most of the changes that happen in our body are remarkable, and scientists are continuing their research to uncover more truth about cannabis.

How does this magic weed work?

In the previous chapter, you learned that cannabis has a remarkable effect on the human body. Most of these effects are obvious and clear. Now the question is, how does it work? Where do these effects originate in the body?

Endogenous cannabinoids

Do you know why marijuana has such an effect on us? Well, it is a surprise that our own body produces chemical components similar to cannabis. These components are known as endogenous cannabinoids (otherwise referred as endocannabinoids). The endocannabinoids in our body regulate many functions, such as blood pressure, the growth of bones, sleep, immune responses, etc. Your body is healthy and well balanced when all these different endocannabinoids work together properly. But when there is an imbalance in these endocannabinoid activities, our body gets affected with various conditions.

Cannabinoid Receptors

Endocannabinoids make use of their biological effects when they bind to the cannabinoid receptors. They primarily act like switches to all the changes in the bodily functions such as appetite, response to pain, blood pressure, etc. Recent studies have confirmed that these cannabinoid receptors are mostly found in many parts of the brain, immune system and various other organs in the body. Endocannabinoids and their cannabinoid receptors together form the endocannabinoid system. This system plays a fundamental role in the basic physiology of every primitive organism on the planet.

When plant cannabinoids meet endocannabinoid

The cannabinoids derived from plants (cannabis) bind to the endocannabinoid receptors to stimulate responses, which are usually regulated by the endocannabinoid system. As mentioned earlier, the cannabinoid receptors are distributed all over the human body. When you consume cannabis, the human body displays specific effects based on the cannabinoid receptor it reacts with. Not all cannabinoids bind directly to the receptors in the body. They might just influence the way other cannabinoids bind.

Most of the cannabinoid receptors are found mainly in the immune system and central nervous system. This is why cannabis is mostly used to treat medical conditions related to immune system or nervous system. For example, multiple sclerosis is the pain with neurologic origin while conditions such as inflammation, rheumatism are due to lack of immunity. However, more researches and clinical trials are necessary to translate the effects into the development of workable medicine.

Restoring the balance

When you use cannabis for recreational purpose, you are intentionally disturbing the balance in your body to enjoy the pleasurable intoxicating experience. On the contrary, when you use cannabis to treat certain medical conditions, the cannabinoids in the cannabis might partly restore the balance again. This is because your body is already out of balance due to the medical condition.

This will help you to look at the differences in using cannabis for medicinal and recreational uses.

Does CBD work for recreational purposes similar to THC?

People who use marijuana for recreational purpose mostly do it for handling stress and anxiety. Therefore, the importance of CBD for these people is advantageous. The ability of CBD to act as a counterweight to THC is one of the many splendid things that amuse people. The best part is – CBD can help produce a more balanced and smoother high.

When people who use cannabis for recreational purpose talk about negative experience, it is mostly due to anxiety and paranoid feeling. The weed you get in the market today can be extremely potent due to the THC (they don't even mention the concentrates). When too much THC goes into the body, it can trigger negative alterations in the mood. CBD can help pump the breaks by hindering the toxicity of THC for people who are either sensitive to THC or people who get too high.

This is a pretty unique mechanism, which works under the entourage effect. There are many edibles, strains, and concentrates that have a combination of a healthy CBD dose with high THC quantity. This is necessary as the CBD in the product can work as an antidote to THC by countering the strong stress-inducing effects of THC. This results in a smooth and well-balanced high.

The 1:1 strains and products with a balanced blend of CBD and THC are quite popular among cannabis users (for a recreational purpose).

Is Cannabidiol the future of healing?

The researches and studies were done on Cannabidiol as an efficient and safe medicine so far seem to be showing a promising future for healing purposes. CBD is one of the most incredible compounds in the natural world due to the following reasons:

- Ability to fight back against the most severe and deadly diseases
- Can be used as a wellness supplement which is gentle on the body

The cannabis industry is getting more innovative because of the super component Cannabidiol (CBD). A plant that cannot get you high is now a key player in today's cannabis revolution.

Medical Cannabis and the diseases it can help treat

Since the 19th and 20th centuries, Marijuana has been used as an important botanical medicine. The Cannabidiol (CBD) content in marijuana has claimed to be the potential universal remedy, as it has helped to heal many diseases. The plant cannabinoids interact with the natural cannabinoid receptors in your body's cell membranes. When a cannabinoid activates another cannabinoid receptor, the psychoactive and therapeutic properties of marijuana get into action.

Cannabinoid receptors play a major role in the functioning of the human body, which includes immunity, growth, appetite, metabolism, pain, anxiety, etc. Dr. Allan Frankel from California has successfully treated numerous patients using medical marijuana for less than a decade now. He is an internist who is certified by the board. He has seen tumors vanish in some of his patients who were given 40 to 60 milligrams of CBD in a day. These patients don't go through any other therapy apart from cannabis.

Medical cannabis can be used to treat the following medical conditions:

- Post-traumatic stress disorder (PTSD)
- Mood disorders
- Seizures
- Multiple sclerosis
- Parkinson's disease
- Dystonia and various other degenerative neurological disorders
- Anxiety

CBD works as a first-rate painkiller while Cannabis oil can heal sunburn overnight when applied on the affected area.

It is complicated to understand the neurological effects of CBD as it interacts with a wide variety of receptors. Disorders such as anxiety and addiction are highly complex as they are the result of an imbalance in multiple receptor systems and certain neural networks in the brain. CBD has multi-targeted effects which are often complex to understand. This can be the potential reason for it to help in treating complex disorders. Researchers are continuing with their ongoing studies to understand the complexity and reveal the complete scope of CBD and its healing potential.

Chapter Four: How to Use?

Are you stepping into the world of cannabinoids for the first time? Are you overwhelmed by the variety of different CBD products available in the market? Well, not to worry! You might have already heard about the natural benefits of CBD and would have always wanted to add that to your wellness regimen. But the problem you would most probably be facing is – how to use CBD?

The legal issues on using CBD will also add on to the confusion. Almost all the CBD products derived from hemp are available across all the fifty US states. You don't even need a prescription for the same! But this is not the case with medical cannabis (marijuana). You will need to first understand the laws in your state before you get your hands on medical cannabis. But don't worry; there is a much simpler solution! Go for legal CBD products from medical marijuana dispensaries and authenticated online retail stores. Any CBD product with less than 1% (0.3% to be accurate) THC composition is legal!

The growing demand for CBD has resulted in the introduction of a wide range of varieties in the CBD products – they come in many forms such as capsules, vapes, liquids, cream, tinctures, etc. You get quite a lot of options. All you need to do is to choose the best ones that would suit your lifestyle and needs! The best part of CBD is it doesn't get you high (as mentioned earlier!). This has led to a string of people queuing behind the said component – health experts, scientists, and medical cannabis patients. CBD-rich products are used to treat various medical conditions, such as cancer, diabetes, rheumatoid arthritis, cardiovascular disease, antibiotic-resistant infection, schizophrenia, chronic pain, Crohn's, PTSD, anxiety, multiple sclerosis and the list goes on...

The scientists now refer CBD as a promising compound, as it can provide a whole lot of therapeutic benefits. They are digging into the details of its biological and physiological functionalities. More than enough clinical studies and preclinical research has already proved that CBD has the following qualities:

- Anti-inflammatory
- Antidepressant
- Anti-tumor
- Anti-oxidant
- Anticonvulsant
- Anti-psychotic
- Neuroprotective

CBD has the ability to remove the beta-amyloid plaque (reason for Alzheimer's) from brain cells and change the expression of gene cells.

CBD-rich cannabis strains were discovered accidentally in North California in 2009 where few certified patients had the permission to access medical cannabis legally. This was a beginning for a lab experiment, which involved healing using cannabis that was rich in CBD. It was a breakthrough for the nation when the whole plant-based cannabis oil rich in CBD arrived for therapeutic use. The whole opinion towards cannabis (marijuana) started to change. Today, nobody asks if medical cannabis works but the actual question is *how do I use cannabis for healing my body?*

THC and CBD – the better element

Healing using cannabis is impossible if you ignore either of these two components – CBD (Cannabidiol) and THC (Tetrahydrocannabinol). They are considered as the first couple in cannabis treatment, and they work well together. THC and CBD interact with one another to accentuate each other's healing qualities. CBD amplifies THC's anticancer and painkilling properties while minimizing its psychoactive property. It doesn't stop here – CBD diminishes the adverse effects (increased heartbeat and anxiety) caused by high THC content.

When CBD and THC are present in adequate amounts in the cannabis product, CBD takes up the responsibility of lowering the *feeling of getting high* caused by THC while extending the duration of its effects. A patient who has used CBD-rich cannabis describes the experience as *relaxing but not getting a stoned feeling*.

Cannabis with more of CBD and less of THC is found to work well with patients affected by metabolic, cardiovascular and liver disorders. This is because THC is not much effective to these issues whereas when it comes to stimulating neurogenesis (creation of new brain cells) both CBD and THC play their part well.

Best ways to consume CBD

It is important to consume cannabis which is rich in CBD in proper dosage – should be optimal for a particular duration to ensure you don't get any unwanted side effects. You can get cannabis flower varieties that are rich in CBD from medical marijuana dispensaries for vaping or smoking. But most of the patients prefer to use cannabis oil concentrates, as they are not too comfortable with inhalable products.

Though the US Federal law bans cannabis, it is possible to use measurable doses of potent cannabis (high on CBD level) in various forms (other than smoking). Cannabis oil products that are rich in CBD can be taken orally or under the tongue (in the form of tinctures, edibles, gel caps, lozenges, and tinctures) or applied on the affected areas. You can also heat the concentrated cannabis oil extracts and inhale it through a vape pen.

Inhaling is good if you are looking to treat sensitive and delicate symptoms that need immediate remedy. The effect of CBD can be experienced with a minute and can last for few hours. When you administer cannabis oil rich in CBD orally, the effect can last for more than four hours. But the beginning of the effects is slow (mostly in 30 to 90 minutes) when compared to inhaling the oil.

Different ways to consume CBD

- Ingest CBD
- Hold under the tongue
- Vaping
- Chew as a gum
- Mix with your food or drink
- Apply topically
- Wash or condition hair using CBD

Ingest CBD

The best way to consume CBD is to simply swallow the pure CBD oil. Most people commonly ingest CBD oil by swallowing as it goes through the digestive system. The liver metabolizes the oil that helps in delivering the active compounds into the body's bloodstream.

You can also hold the oil on your tongue before swallowing the CBD oil. The oil comes in different varieties – filtered, decarboxylated and non-decarboxylated. You can also ingest CBD by swallowing CBD oil capsules on a daily basis.

Hold under the tongue

This is another commonly used method for consuming CBD. You can apply and hold the CBD oil under the tongue. The mucus membranes in the mouth will absorb CBD and the active compounds found in the CBD oil. Consuming CBD through this method is faster than the earlier one as the CBD, and the natural constituents found in the oil bypasses the digestive system and liver metabolism process and directly reaches the bloodstream.

Vaping

Vaping CBD has become quite popular in the last one year among people who consume cannabis for wellness. This method of consuming CBD is good and friendly for the lungs. While inhaling the CBD oil through vape pens, the CBD and the other cannabinoids are absorbed directly by the lungs and spread into the bloodstream.

Start simple when you are going to vape CBD for the first time. The easiest way is to use a CBD vaporizer pen. How do I use it? It is an effortless method – charge the base, run the cartridge of CBD oil onto the pen, press the button to turn it on and inhale using its mouthpiece. When you use the vape for the first time, the cartridge will already be packaged with the CBD oil. You can refill the CBD oil cartridges when it is over.

Chew as a gum

This is a simple and enjoyable way to consume CBD. Chew a piece of CBD gum after your morning coffee. Or maybe you can use it as a mouth freshener after your lunch or dinner. You get your daily intake of CBD and at the same time enjoy the experience. A piece of CBD chew gum can have 10 gm of CBD along with the other ingredients.

Mix with your food or drink

Blend the CBD with your favorite food or beverages. This is the easiest way of the lot. When you mix the CBD with the wholesome, healthy food you have prepared, you are giving it an option to get absorbed well into your body. Your food will have the fatty acids that are required by your body. These fatty acids act as a carrier for the cannabinoids to pass through the body for better and faster processing.

You can make any food you consume as our personalized CBD edible. Salads, smoothies, ice cream, coffee, etc. – it can be anything of your choice.

Apply Topically

CBD products can also be applied to your skin directly. When they are topically applied, they get absorbed by the skin and interact with the cell membranes near the skin surface. They don't enter into the bloodstream in this case. Topical CBD products come in either of these forms - creams, lotions, ointments, salves, etc. The CBD oil derived from hemp contains many fatty acids, nutrients, proteins, vitamins along with the CBD and other cannabinoids. These play a major role in improving your skin's health condition.

Wash or condition hair using CBD

There are many varieties of CBD oil conditioners and shampoos available in the market. Most of them are derived from organic hemp oil, which helps to strengthen your hair roots and give you a healthy scalp.

Chapter Five: CBD for Chronic Pain

Many are turning towards medical cannabis to get away from risky and addictive painkillers. Opioids is said to have caused a lot of deaths due to over dose in the United States. Cannabis is now looked at as an effective alternative to these dangerous painkillers. The THC in the weed helps in reducing the pain due to its psychoactive property. However, a recent study in 2015 revealed that Cannabidiol (CBD) is also a potential reliever of acute and chronic pain. Researchers administered CBD with morphine for chronic pain conditions, and surprisingly it worked well. CBD counteracted the risky side effects of morphine and helped to treat chronic pain with long-term benefits.

The natural remedy, which comes in the form of CBD, is now considered to be an effective pain management solution. This is crucial for people who are suffering from chronic and neuropathic pain or pain that lasts for months. Do you know what the worst thing about chronic pain is? It can be treated but cannot be cured! The most commonly used medical treatments for chronic pain are steroids, narcotics (i.e., opioids) and nerve blocks. Unfortunately, all these carry dangerous side effects and addiction. There are certain drugs such as ibuprofen and Aspirin, which can get dangerous when used on a regular basis. These non-steroidal anti-inflammatory drugs (NSAIDs) have killed close to 15000 approximately.

When compared to these drugs, CBD is entirely safe, non-toxic and not addictive. The best part is it is a natural product derived from the plants with minimum or no side effects. CBD can help relieve pain if used continuously. Are you suffering from chronic pain in your back, neck, feet, hand or elsewhere? Well, CBD is your solution!

Chronic pain relief

Both the cannabinoids – CBD and THC are useful for various acute pain conditions. They have proved to work well especially to control neuropathic pain. What is neuropathic pain? It is the chronic pain you feel in the nerves (the ones that are waning), which might also lead to numbness or tingling sensation. They are known as CRPS (Complex Regional Pain Syndrome) and were earlier referred as RSD (Reflex Sympathetic Dystrophy). This type of chronic pain occurs due to peripheral nerve injury or could also be mediated by other factors.

Studies show that it is possible to manage chronic pain by activating CB2 receptors. CBD is helpful in activating CB2 receptors as they are attached to these receptors and help ease the chronic pain. Most of the time, these acute and chronic pains are associated with degenerative conditions like multiple sclerosis, diabetes, and fibromyalgia. How does CBD help here? When CBD is administered, they can target and activate the glycine receptors (located in the spinal cord and brain regions) in the central nervous system. What does CBD exactly do? They reactivate the receptors that are shut down by inflammatory factors like prostaglandins in the body. When the receptors don't work, the sensation of pain increases. CBD reactivates these receptors that result in less pain (decreased pain). This makes CBD an anti-inflammatory agent and helps to kill the pain-inducing effects.

CBD oil can be considered to be an effective pain management method to relieve people from chronic pain. You don't get addicted when you use CBD regularly, and it isn't toxic too.

Multiple sclerosis

This autoimmune disease affects the entire body through the brain and nerves. The most common symptoms in this disease are muscle spasms – which causes constant pain to many. Though we don't have many clinical studies on humans to confirm that CBD can lessen the pain in MS, many who have used CBD oil have stated that they did notice a reduction in the symptoms. The levels of spasticity were considerably low when CBD was consumed regularly.

Generic acute pain

A lot of trials and studies were conducted to check if medical cannabis could cure chronic pain in adults. A study conducted by the Journal of Experimental Medicine could prove that regular CBD usage noticed a reduction in inflammation and pain. They could conclude with substantial evidence that medical cannabis could indeed work for chronic pain. The best part was the subjects (ones affected by general chronic pain) didn't build any tolerance to the CBD effects and therefore didn't require the need to increase the dosage.

Dosage, Side effects, and Benefits

The United States Food and Drug Administration (FDA) has not regulated the use of CBD. Therefore, dosages can be followed as stated in the Directions to Use section of the label. But you need to be cautious depending on your medical condition. Some companies advise high dosages while some recommend lesser dosages.

The dosage can be between 2.5 to 20 milligrams orally for 25 days to treat chronic pain. It is always advisable to start with lower dosages (2.5 mg) when you start. You can gradually increase the dosage in few days.

It is advisable to contact your medical practitioner if you don't see positive effects of the dosage or if you see any adverse effects.

CBD doesn't have any harmful side effects in most people as people mostly tolerate them. The *Cannabis and Cannabinoid Research* published its results on a review of the most commonly found side effects of CBD:

- Diarrhea
- Weight loss or Weight gain
- Tiredness
- Appetite issues.

If you are planning to take CBD oil along with your other medications, it is best to check with the doctor as the medications can react with CBD. Avoid using CBD oil for children unless a doctor recommends it. There are not many clinical studies on what effect CBD might have on the developing brain of a child. It is strictly not recommended for nursing mothers or pregnant women.

The most commonly noticed *benefits* of CBD on Chronic Pain are:

- It helps in relaxing the body muscles
- Good sleep
- Relief from anxiety
- Anti-inflammatory
- It helps to reduce the fear of touch in some patients
- Reduces depression
- Works on PTSD
- Non-psychotropic (Not a drug that affects the mental health)
- You don't feel like you are taking medicine.

Studies and Researches

There was a study conducted in 2014, which investigated the therapeutic potential of CBD in treating CIPN. The result was positive. To know more:
https://www.ncbi.nlm.nih.gov/pubmed/24117398

Another study was conducted on how cannabinoids can help relieve neuropathic pain the same year. It stated – *"The endocannabinoid system has been elucidated over the last several years, demonstrating a significant interface with pain homeostasis. Exogenous (plant-based) cannabinoids have been demonstrated to be effective in a range of experimental neuropathic pain models, and there is mounting evidence for therapeutic use in human neuropathic pain conditions."* To know more, https://www.ncbi.nlm.nih.gov/pubmed/25160710

Similarly, a lot of studies were conducted between 2010 and 2015 to check how effective CBD is to relieve chronic pain.

When you are looking to formulate the use of CBD for a particular disease (chronic pain), it is important to use it regularly for maximum benefit. It should first be used as a defensive method to regulate the base of your system. Maintenance is important, so you need to look at it as a dietary supplement.

Chapter Six: Anxiety and Seizures

CBD products are reported to be effective in treating anxiety and many other neurological conditions by people who had used it on themselves (self-experiment). According to them, retail CBD products with lower levels of other cannabinoids are said to work on anxiety-related disorders. CBD has been specifically used to treat PTSD, anxiety and other conditions related to brain illness.

As per the Department of Health and Human Services US Patent,

"No signs of toxicity or serious side effects have been observed following chronic administration of cannabidiol to healthy volunteers (Cunha et al., Pharmacology 21:175-185, 1980), even in large acute doses of 700 mg/day (Consroe et al., Pharmacol. Biochem. Behav. 40:701-708, 1991)"

Anxiety

Anxiety is not something all of us wish for, but it is a critical adaptive response that usually helps us to cope with the threats for our safety. If you are anxious about something, it means the mind has recognized a potential threat, which needs to be warded off. But anxiety is not completely a negative sign; it can help motivate you to do better in improving the current position. For instance, to work harder, to concentrate on your relationship, to save money for traveling, etc.

However, the issue begins when we don't handle these natural responses properly. They get overboard and start to show a serious impact on our daily routine (work, relationship, etc.). This ultimately leads to anxiety-related conditions that require medical attention. *Stress kills!* And it is 100 percent true.

There have been numerous evidences from human experiments, clinical trials and epidemiological studies that suggest CBD to have strong anti-anxiety properties. When CBD is administered with the right dosage, it emerges as a safe and beneficial option to treat various anxiety-related disorders, which includes:

- OCD (Obsessive Compulsive Disorder)
- PTSD (Post Traumatic Stress Disorder)
- Depression (Mild to moderate)
- Panic disorder
- Social phobia
  GAD (Generalized Anxiety Disorder)

How CBD reduces anxiety?

There have been numerous human studies that show CBD works effectively in reducing anxiety.

A double-blind study was conducted by Brazilian researchers on patients who were affected by generalized social anxiety. The participants who had consumed CBD reported a major decrease in their anxiety levels. Researchers had confirmed the same by validating these patients' individual reports after carrying out brain scans. The cerebral blood flow patterns in these scans confirmed that the CBD's anti-anxiety effect had indeed benefited them.

There was another study where researchers had asked the patients suffering from Social Anxiety Disorder to perform a public speaking test. They were able to note a visible difference in them after consuming the CBD. The participants reported feeling less anxious at their simulated test. This finding was supported by the objective anxiety indicators (blood pressure and heart rate).

It was then concluded that CBD, in fact, helped to reduce cognitive impairment, discomfort, and anxiety during their speech performances. But the patients who were asked to have placebo reported higher anxiety, discomfort, and cognitive impairment.

There have been more human studies of patients (with and without anxiety) to validate the efficiency of CBD as an effective anti-anxiety therapeutic cure. Large RCTs (randomized control trials) have been conducted to study the long-term effects CBD can offer. Researchers and medical experts are looking to confirm if CBD would be a favorable safety option when compared to the current set of drugs used (to control anxiety).

Seizures

Parents who have kids affected by epileptic-based seizures or non-epileptic seizures are looking at CBD as a magic herb given by nature. CBD has been effective in treating seizures – especially in children. I hope you remember the news on a child who was affected by constant seizures magically able to stop them by using CBD tinctures. The child had probably taken tons of medicines to stop the seizures, but none of them worked. Finally, CBD did it – no more seizures. Is this even possible? To an extent, yes! There have been many studies that evaluated CBD's role on different types of seizures.

Epilepsy is a seizure disorder condition, which affects more than fifty million people globally. Unfortunately, these seizures cannot be cured completely but only controlled. Many medicines are required to keep the seizures under control. Anticonvulsants, sedatives, painkillers, nerve pain medication, etc. are some of the medications that are normally prescribed by the medical practitioners.

The issue with all these medications is they come with a host of side effects that can completely disturb and ruin one's life routine. Sometimes the patients are addicted to few of the drugs prescribed to them. This is the main reason for people (especially children) to use CBD, as it is a natural plant-based solution, which doesn't come with any complications. CBD can reduce the number of seizures with minimum to no side effects. Irrespective of the issue - general epilepsy, seizure or specific disorders (Dravet Syndrome), CBD can come to your rescue.

The researchers wanted to confirm this, and they searched through the entire research databases thoroughly for relevant published as well as unpublished studies. They looked at the papers, to check on the potential impact of using CBD as an additional healing method to their existing medical treatment on epilepsy seizures. They could find 91 studies. Six of them were clinical trials that involved 555 patients, and 30 of them were observational studies that involved 2865 patients. All these findings were included in their review. Almost all the participants had epilepsy (rare forms), which didn't respond to their usual treatment. The average age of the participants was sixteen.

The collective investigation of the clinical trial disclosed that CBD was effective when compared to the placebo drug. They could reduce the frequency of the seizures by more than 50 percent thereby improving the kid's quality of life. There were few cases where seizures were completely eradicated. Drowsiness and dizziness were the commonly noted side effects.

Similarly, the collective data from 17 observational studies showed more than 50 percent drop in the seizure frequency in half of the patients. Around one in ten had no seizures at all. Finally, the researchers concluded that CBD is effective for seizures and the following review has been published online (Journal of Neurology Neurosurgery & Psychiatry)

"Pharmaceutical grade CBD as adjuvant treatment in pediatric onset drug-resistant epilepsy may reduce seizure frequency, Existing [randomized controlled trial] evidence is mostly

in pediatric samples with rare and severe epilepsy syndromes; [randomized controlled trials] examining other syndromes and cannabinoids are needed."

More Studies and Researches

15 patients who had general epilepsy in timely interval were divided into 2 groups. A double-bind procedure was followed where each patient was administered with Placebo or CBD on a regular basis. Patients who were given CBD had shown significant improvement in their condition. To know more details, visit https://www.ncbi.nlm.nih.gov/pubmed/7413719

There was another study conducted in 2014 to check how effective plant-based cannabinoids are on seizures. The result showed that the endocannabinoids were altered to reduce epileptic seizures. To know more, visit https://www.ncbi.nlm.nih.gov/pubmed/25346637.

Chapter Seven: Fibromyalgia

People who are affected by Fibromyalgia have been trying to find an alternative healing method to ease the pain for many years now. Thanks to the entry of non-psychoactive CBD (Cannabidiol), most people are looking at this natural plant-based component as a potential remedy to Fibromyalgia and many other similar medical conditions. In recent years, CBD has brought hope to people affected by Fibromyalgia. The CBD oil or extract is able to provide relief and ease the pain the natural way. It also helps to keep the body from chemical reactions and serious side effects caused by the usual medicines.

Fibromyalgia patients who had tried CBD as an alternative medicine and found their source of recovery had published their inspirational stories. These stories have influenced and encouraged more people with similar health disorder to try CBD. Though Fibromyalgia cannot be cured, CBD helps to ease the pain and reduce the discomfort that occurs in the body. CBD makes the pain bearable and less noticeable.

Effect of CBD on Fibromyalgia pain

What is Fibromyalgia? It is a chronic pain disorder, which causes widespread muscle pain and tenderness. The musculoskeletal pain can cause cognitive issues and fatigue. There is no permanent cure for this disorder. All the treatment options focus on managing the pain, i.e., reducing the pain and making it bearable.

Studies have shown that CBD can be an effective solution to reduce inflammation and reduce symptoms of chronic pain. It is also being considered as an alternative to opioid drugs as they are highly addictive to the patients. As mentioned earlier, the FDA has not yet approved any CBD-based treatment as a regulated treatment option.

People who have used CBD oil for their fibromyalgia issues have reported to experience a decrease in pain. They claim the pain to be bearable and add that it has also helped in getting rid of fatigue (a common symptom in fibromyalgia). CBD can be applied as a gel or cream on the pain-affected area or all over the body. They can also be orally administered as oil or tincture.

The reach of this miracle plant-based cannabinoid has extended beyond individual experiences and social media articles. Global media outlets such as The Wall Street Journal, CNN, and Men's Health have featured about CBD Oil (Elixinol) in their magazines.

Studies and Researches

Multiple studies have been conducted to check the ability of CBD oil and its effectiveness on various medical conditions including Fibromyalgia.

There was a study published in 2011 that was conducted by Fiz et al. – Various dosages of cannabis were administered to 28 patients affected by Fibromyalgia. They were tested for pain levels after they had consumed the medical cannabis. The participants who had CBD reported that they felt a decrease in pain. The Visual Analogue Scale (VAS) scoring for analysis confirmed the reports. The scientists who had conducted the research wrote their final report - *"the use of cannabis was associated with beneficial effects on some FM symptoms."*

Russo EB had conducted a study in 2009 to test the efficacy of cannabinoids on Fibromyalgia and migraines. The result concluded that Fibromyalgia, Migraine, IBS and other related conditions that displayed similar biochemical, pathophysiological and clinical patterns might be treated with cannabinoid-based medicines.

Carrie Anton from Minnesota had blogged her personal experience on easing pain caused by Fibromyalgia using CBD. She had tried the CBD oil, and within three days she could see the difference in her pain symptoms. The best part is the oil was CBD-rich with little THC. To know more, check https://fibromyalgianewstoday.com/2017/11/03/seeking-fibro-pain-relief-cbd-oil-my-experience/

These are only a few cases that prove the effectiveness of CBD on Fibromyalgia, but when you dig deeper, you will be able to find so many other success stories, clinical trials and personal experiences.

The five best CBD oils for Fibromyalgia are – Elixinol, CBDessence.net, CBDpure. PureKana and Greenroadsworld.

People who are suffering from severe pain and serious discomforts of Fibromyalgia can definitely choose CBD oil as the safest natural alternative to the conventional medicines.

Chapter Eight: CBD to Reduce Opioids

Ongoing research on CBD has shown that this non-psychoactive component might help treat patients who are addicted to opioids. What is opioid? An opioid is a substance used in medical industry as anesthesia and to relieve people from pain. These act on the opioid receptors in the brain to give morphine-like effects. Most people get addicted to opioid drugs during the course of time. CBD is said to reduce the addiction towards opioids and also treat acute, chronic pain.

The overdoses of opioid in the medical industry have become a sign of concern. It is so bad that around three times as many people die every year from opioid overdoses in the United States. This is indeed more than gun-related homicides. As per the Centers for Disease Control and Prevention (CDC), around 33,000 deaths have been confirmed due to opioid overdose while gun-related homicides caused 11,000 deaths.

Opioid-related deaths have gone up to 400 percent in the last twelve years. 2016 witnessed the death of around 19,000 people due to opioids in the United States. This means around 52 people die on an average per day and this is a very dangerous figure. President Trump declared an opioids emergency in 2017. He has extended the public health emergency declaration for opioids again this year (2018.)

The only apparent solution to this dangerous outbreak of opioid addiction is CBD. CBD is the natural solution that can help people from this addiction and give them a good quality of life. New studies show that medical cannabis is indeed our best answer to this crisis.

Role of cannabis in Opioids and Chronic Pain

Why is opioid given to patients? To relieve them from acute pain! So, the underlying source of the opioid crisis is the chronic pain. Since chronic pain is severe and serious, it requires constant medication to treat and keep it under control. Opioids do provide a solution to these patients by easing the pain, making it bearable and providing relief to the uncomfortable feeling. But the problem here is – they are awfully addictive.

Opioids work well for the chronic pain experienced by the patient to recover from the surgery or other disorders. Constant doses in small quantity over a long period of time can get the patient hooked. So, when the prescription is finally done, and opioid is no longer needed, the patient finds it unable to resist himself from having the drug. The doctor would definitely not encourage continuing the opioid drug, and so people turn to other means to procure the drug. This is when the addiction becomes quite dangerous.

Cannabis can act as an alternative medicine to opioid for pain relief. A Major review of cannabis has shown that the magic herb is a natural form of cure for many medical conditions. Cannabis had provided the best relief for chronic pain in a particular study. There was another study that showed CBD to have a long-lasting effect than methadone. Methadone has to be regularly administered, but the lasting effect of CBD provides a more sustainable mode of healing. The best part of CBD is – it doesn't numb the patient's mind or get him hooked. Therefore, it is definitely better to use CBD to treat chronic pain instead of administering the opioid-based drugs.

Block the addiction

Opioids trigger a reward pathway for the patients, which get consistent with time. This results in the patient getting hooked. As time goes by, it is no longer about the pain but about the reward pathway. The opioids force the brain to one specific pathway – they maintain a feeling of *it-is-difficult-to-get-payoff* of addiction. When you stop the reward pathway, the addiction naturally subsides. CBD does exactly this!

A new research shows that CBD naturally restrains the reward-facilitating effect of not just the opioid drugs but also works on other intoxicative behavior such as smoking, alcoholism, etc. CBD has the potential to help numerous people to get off from their addictive behavior as the same neural pathway causes almost all addictions. CBD is definitely the safest solution to help people with opiate withdrawal and to curtail the epidemic deaths.

Case Study

Richard (name changed) broke a disc in his spine when he was 34. This resulted in acute back pain, and he was prescribed OxyContin for pain relief. Richard had taken the drug for a year, but the doctor had canceled his prescription as he suspected him to be misusing the drug. By then, Richard was addicted to OxyContin and had started to find other ways to access the drug. This included stealing money from his family.

When he was 37, he had lost his career, family and was almost homeless, as he had nearly become a criminal to continue with his addiction. He was addicted to the opiate (OxyContin) for close to seven years. Soon, he started to work his way out of the addiction mode. He started withdrawing from the drug, and this resulted in severe depression.

To escape from his depression, he began to smoke weed (marijuana) as suggested by his friend. Marijuana helped to lessen his pain (back pain), but the urge to continue with OxyContin was still there. Richard then tried CBD three years back (around 2015) and thankfully in Canada (the place where he lives), CBD is legal for medicinal use. It can be bought in pill form from medical dispensaries.

After he started to take CBD, his cravings for the opium reduced and he could feel the difference. It was a new beginning for him. Today, he takes one CBD capsule (33 mg) per day. He had reported to MensHealth.com that the Cannabidiol helped him to get back to work, to meet people without getting anxious, etc.

Inference

There are many cases similar to Richard's and almost every one of them had reported CBD as their lifesaver. This cannabinoid had given a new lease of life to many people who have been suffering from acute and chronic pain. Opioid addiction is officially considered to be the main cause of fatal drug overdose in the United States.

Multiple studies have shown that medical marijuana, which is rich in CBD, is the only best alternative to opioids like Vicodin, OxyContin, etc. Since it doesn't get you *high*, medical experts are looking at CBD to rework the neural pathways in the addict's brain to help with withdrawal symptoms and reduce cravings.

The Scripps Research Institute in San Diego has provided evidence in their new research that CBD could work as an effective treatment for any substance addiction.

Majority of the people have already started to refer CBD as a miracle drug that helps in improving the health and wellness of the body. The benefits are not restricted only to the medical arena but extend to the areas of food, beauty, fitness, etc.

You don't have to use CBD on a daily basis for it to be effective as it is long lasting.

Chapter Nine: CBD for Cancer

Multiple studies have been carried out to conclude on CBD's efficacy as a healing aid for cancer. The preliminary results also confirm that CBD can kill cancer cells. Scientists have reported that it is possible for CBD to slow down the growth of cancer and tumor cells. In some cases, it has also been the reason for the death of certain cancerous cells. Clinical trials can be found on CBD's usage to mitigate cancer in humans. However, we still need more studies to establish and confirm the efficiency of CBD to treat cancer-related symptoms.

The US Food and Drug Administration (FDA) has still not approved Cannabis for the treatment of any cancer-related symptoms or for the side effects caused by cancer treatment. The following two cannabinoids have been approved by the FDA to treat nausea and vomiting caused by chemotherapy in patients:

- Nabilone
- Dronabinol

But this should be used only if the patient doesn't respond to the standard conventional therapy.

Does CBD fight the cancer cells?

CBD moves towards the CB2 receptors that are responsible for activating the body's immune system. These CB2 receptors are found in the spleen (an abdominal organ). CBD mimics the biochemical processing to the body's Anandamide, which then activates the CB2 receptors. What does this mean? It means your body can use CBD and the Anandamide interchangeably for the immune purpose. So, when your body is affected by external injury (illness, wound, etc.) or internal disorder (stress, depression, etc.), it tends to demand more Anandamide then the body can produce. In this case, your body activates the mimetic CBD.

If there is temporary stress to the body, the healing aid will be temporary. But if the stress remains (in the case of stress caused by cancer), the CBD provides a constant pressure of a regulating agent on the homeostatic (internal) system. The thing is, once the CBD moves towards CB2 receptors, it looks out for the cancer cells or cancer causing cells and destroys them. Studies have proved that CBD can kill the cancer cells directly without getting the mediators of the immune system involved. The reason for this is – CBD can take control of the lipoxygenase pathway to hinder the growth of cancer cells and tumors directly.

Using CBD to relieve cancer is advantageous in many ways, and the most important of them is there are no side effects and the fact that you don't get high. Apart from these, there are a series of positive effects on cancer-affected patients. They are:

- Triggers the death of cancerous cells
- Prevents harmful cell division
- Stops the growth of tumors in the new blood vessels
- Slows down the spread of cancer cells all through the body and also gradually reduces them.
- Speeds up the autophagy process

These effects are possible because CBD interacts with the CB2 receptors. But as mentioned earlier, more studies are required to confirm the effectiveness of CBD as an alternative or complementary cancer healing aid.

Things to remember

Cancer is a dangerous and deadly disease. If the right treatment is not given at the right time, it can prove fatal to the patient's health condition. It is, therefore, crucial to take a calculated medical decision after consulting your doctor.

Though CBD doesn't cause any side effects, it is better to keep your doctor informed on your choice so that it will help him to monitor the progress.

Clinical trials

The CAM on PubMed database maintained by the National Institutes of Health doesn't carry any new or ongoing trials of cannabis with regards to cancer treatment on humans. Earlier clinical trials had helped to study the efficacy of cannabis and its cannabinoids in treating the side effects of cancers.

Cancer

- CBD was used by mouth to treat tumors (solid) that had come back after surgery
- Combination of two cannabinoids (CBD and delta-9-THC) was given with temozolomide in the form of an oral spray to treat glioblastoma multiforme (chronic)
- Patients who had undergone stem cell transplantation (allogeneic hematopoietic) were given CBD to treat their acute graft-vs-host disease.

Chemotherapy

- Cannabis was used in an inhaled form to treat nausea and vomiting caused by

chemotherapy. Ten small trials were conducted on this with a combination of various chemotherapy agents and study methods. Not enough information is found to interpret the findings.
- A double-blinded clinical trial in Spain used Oral spray with delta-9-THC and CBD to treat vomiting and nausea caused by Chemotherapy. Placebo drugs were also given for few to check the difference.

Chapter Ten: CBD for Health

The revolutionary CBD research and its natural benefits have already encouraged many people to include CBD oil into their routine to get relief from their existing medical conditions. It doesn't stop here! CBD can also be used as a natural dietary supplement to people who would want to keep their health and wellness intact. The botanical properties in the CBD help provide these benefits naturally.

The natural cannabinoids found in the cannabis plants – hemp and marijuana interact with the body's native ECS system to promote health and balance. CBD is the natural non-psychoactive component that can work well for better health. The CBD concentrate derived from the seeds and stalks of the hemp plant can be used in the form of oil or other forms.

How does CBD promote to improve health?

CBD and other traces of cannabinoids found in the CBD oil (derived from hemp or marijuana) begin to interact with the endocannabinoid system (ECS) of the body. As mentioned earlier, the ECS found in every living organism (mostly) regulates a wide series of body's functionalities (immune, hormone, growth, sleep, mood, appetite, etc.). It is the job of the ECS to keep these functions in control by providing the necessary balance.

Your body and mind are completely hale and healthy when the ECS does its work properly. The ECS ensures that all our body cells stick to their optimal performance. When an external force disturbs the body's cell and pushes it to go out of control, the ECS is summoned to make the required adjustments to bring the cell back into its balanced state. This is referred as homeostasis (internal balance).

The ECS gets benefitted by cannabinoids like CBD when it interacts with the cannabinoid receptors in the immune system, central nervous system, and peripheral system. It helps to stimulate the ECS by encouraging it to keep all the functions at its optimum performance and balance.

People who are healthy can regulate their body for steady health and wellness by consuming CBD as a dietary supplement.

Dietary necessities provided by CBD

Hemp-derived CBD oil can help support the health and wellness of your body. The oil provides the body with nutrients that are not sufficiently available in today's diet (including the healthy people).

CBD oil is said to be the natural source of essential minerals and vitamins, such as:

- Vitamin E
- Vitamin C
- B Complex Vitamins
- Magnesium
- Calcium

Apart from these, CBD oil is also a source of flavonoids, protein, fatty acids and terpenes. These nutrients help your body to function efficiently.

CBD need not be restricted only to people who have medical conditions. They can serve as a natural supplement to everyone who is looking to have a healthy and well-balanced life. The nutritional content of hemp combined with the effects of CBD will ensure your body to be a beacon of perfect health.

CBD oil derived from hemp is legally available in all the dispensaries and online retail outlets. CBD oil derived from marijuana will require you to check the legal laws in your area before you take possession of it. But if the composition of THC is less than 1 percent or is 0.3 percent, it is considered legal. Nevertheless, it is still advisable to check the laws to avoid unwanted legal hiccups.

You can add CBD to your daily routine for your physical and mental wellness. Since CBD hemp oil is a nutritional supplement, it can be purchased in all the 50 US states and in 40 countries globally. But to get access to medical cannabis oil, you might need a prescription from the medical practitioner.

Chapter Eleven: Safety and Legal Issues

With more and more people looking at CBD as their favorable option for health, there have been more concerns on the purity and quality of the products. Since there are no regulations imposed by FDA on the CBD products, it becomes all the more important to ensure the CBD oil you purchase is of high quality and is completely legal.

The Drug Enforcement Administration (DEA) has been closely watching the development that has been happening with cannabis and CBD. The non-psychoactive cannabinoid has improved the lives of countless people across the globe. Many medical experts are thinking of it as an alternative medicine to various health disorders (though more studies are needed in this regard). Recently, the DEA had instilled fear in many when they talked about the CBD restrictions (as it is still termed as Schedule 1 drug).

So how is it possible to know if the acquired CBD is legal or not? All you need to do is check the source and label. For instance, Medix CBD, Elixinol, RSHO, Canazall, etc. are legal CBD products and are safe to use across any state in the US.

Don't forget to look at the following three things before you buy CBD oil online:

- THC should be less 0.03%
- CBD oil should be extracted through Decarboxylation process
- Check the third party lab results

Difference between Legal and Illegal CBD oil

- CBD products made from *cannabis* strains are legal in the states where marijuana is considered legal. This is because THC will be on the higher end as it is made from marijuana.
- CBD products derived from *hemp* strains are legal in all the fifty states of the country. But the composition of THC should be 0.3%.
- Though hemp and cannabis are almost similar, the main feature that distinguishes both is the cannabinoid composition. (Hemp will have more CBD, Cannabis (marijuana) will have more THC)
- There are companies that sell hemp oil with little or no cannabinoids as CBD oil. This is illegal.

The consumers should research the company's website to ensure the CBD oil which is being purchased is safe and legal.

Cannabis is legal in fifty percent of the states for medicinal purpose as on date. Another seventeen states approve the use of cannabis products that have high CBD content and low THC content. But again, it should be only for medicinal purpose. These products are available in medical marijuana dispensaries, normal dispensaries, and online retail stores.

The underlying fact is that FDA approves none of these products. The DEA had recently denied two rescheduling petitions on marijuana, i.e., marijuana and hemp are still classified as Schedule 1 drug. However, they are taking steps to smoothen the progress of future research.

Conclusion

We have come to the end of this book. I would like to take this opportunity to thank you once again for choosing this book.

I sincerely hope this book was useful and helped you as a reader to get a clear, in-depth understanding on medical cannabis and its CBD component. This book would have given a detailed description on CBD, its history and the way it works on the human body. The chapters concentrate on various benefits of CBD on our health and wellness.

I hope this book was useful and has helped in answering most of the queries you had in mind.

Thank you and best wishes!

Sources

https://bluebirdbotanicals.com/hemp-cbd-oil-faq/

https://www.projectcbd.org/about/what-cbd

https://hightimes.com/health/cannabidiol-cbd/

https://www.history.com/topics/history-of-marijuana

https://www.deamuseum.org/ccp/cannabis/history.html

https://www.livescience.com/48337-marijuana-history-how-cannabis-travelled-world.html

http://www.ncsm.nl/english/what-is-medicinal-cannabis/how-does-cannabis-work

https://articles.mercola.com/medical-marijuana-uses.aspx

https://www.medicalmarijuanainc.com/first-time-cbd-user-7-ways-can-take-cbd/

https://www.projectcbd.org/guidance/cbd-users-manual

https://www.healthline.com/health/cbd-oil-for-pain#further-research

https://www.medicalnewstoday.com/articles/319475.php

https://drdavidbrady.com/blogs/news/cbd-and-chronic-pain

https://www.honeycolony.com/article/10-benefits-of-cbd-for-chronic-pain/

https://keytocannabis.com/blogs/cannabis/how-to-use-cbd-for-pain-management

https://www.leafly.com/news/health/cbd-for-treating-anxiety

https://www.europeanpharmaceuticalreview.com/news/73449/cbd-epileptic-seizures/

https://keytocannabis.com/blogs/cannabis/cbd-for-seizures-and-epilepsy

https://www.marijuanabreak.com/best-cbd-oils-for-fibromyalgia

https://www.healthline.com/health/cbd-for-fibromyalgia#outlook

https://www.menshealth.com/health/a19607404/marijuana-drug-addiction-cbd-opioid-cocaine-use/

https://haveaheartcc.com/cannabidiol-for-opiate-withdrawal/

https://cbdoilsandedibles.com/cbd-for-cancer/

https://www.cancer.gov/about-cancer/treatment/cam/patient/cannabis-pdq#section/_3

https://www.medicalmarijuanainc.com/heres-cbd-can-help-whether-youre-healthy-not/

https://hightimes.com/sponsored/cbd-oil-legal-high-quality/

Thank you again for downloading this book!

I hope this book was able to help you get some value you were seeking for.

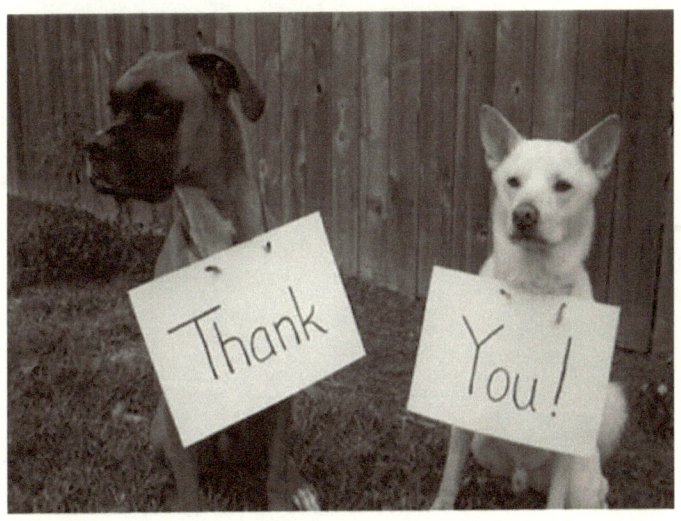

Finally, if you enjoyed this book, **then I'd like to ask you for a favor, would you be kind enough to leave a review for this book on Amazon?** It'd be greatly appreciated!

Thank you and good luck!

www.ingramcontent.com/pod-product-compliance
Lightning Source LLC
Chambersburg PA
CBHW031531210526
45464CB00012B/2445